Thyroid Healing

Heal It With Natural Remedies and Proper Nutrition

(Quick Guide to Learning the Thyroid and Natural Remedies to Heal the Thyroid)

Timothy Ross

Published By **Jackson Denver**

Timothy Ross

Thyroid Healing: Heal It With Natural Remedies and Proper Nutrition (Quick Guide to Learning the Thyroid and Natural Remedies to Heal the Thyroid)

ISBN 978-1-998901-27-2

Legal & Disclaimer

The information contained in this ebook is not designed to replace or take the place of any form of medicine or professional medical advice. The information in this ebook has been provided for educational & entertainment purposes only.

The information contained in this book has been compiled from sources deemed reliable, and it is accurate to the best of the Author's knowledge; however, the Author cannot guarantee its accuracy and validity and cannot be held liable for any errors or omissions. Changes are periodically made to this book. You must consult your doctor or get professional medical advice before using any of the suggested remedies, techniques, or information in this book.

Upon using the information contained in this book, you agree to hold harmless the Author from and against any damages, costs, and expenses, including any legal fees potentially resulting from the application of any of the information provided by this guide. This disclaimer applies to any damages or injury caused by the use and application, whether directly or indirectly, of any advice or information presented, whether for breach of contract, tort, negligence, personal injury, criminal intent, or under any other cause of action.

You agree to accept all risks of using the information presented inside this book. You need to consult a professional medical practitioner in order to ensure you are both able and healthy enough to participate in this program.

Table Of Contents

Chapter 1: The Thyroid Epidemic

The human body is undeniably the maximum complex gadget inside the worldwide, crafted from masses of thousands of small elements that paintings together to keep lifestyles. The endocrine gland is an crucial a part of this gadget, liberating precise chemical materials referred to as "hormones" into the blood. Hormones journey to every a ways flung nook of the frame, appearing vital abilties including metabolism, growth and sexual improvement.

1.1 THE THYROID GLAND

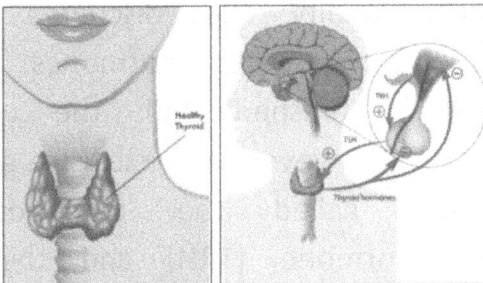

The thyroid gland is a hint butterfly-common organ, determined at the front of the neck. It has lobes that lie on each aspect of the windpipe or trachea. The gland releases 3 important hormones (Calcitonin, thyroxine and triiodothyronine) which might be critical for digestion, muscle manipulate, brain development, temper and bone protection. Triiodothyronine is the activated shape of thyroxine, however, now not all thyroxine gets activated. Like the entirety else inside the body, hormone tiers also are regulated primarily based on need.

Two important regions inside the mind referred to as the hypothalamus and pituitary modify the discharge and activation of thyroid hormones. This manage is finished with the useful resource of however each exclusive set of hormones called the thyrotrophin-releasing-hormone (TRH) and thyroid-stimulating hormone (TSH). TSH acts like a messenger a number of the mind and the thyroid gland. When the mind detects depleting degrees of thyroid hormones, it sends within the TSH to tell the thyroid gland to provide more. In a healthy man or woman, this feedback loop works flawlessly, usually generating simply the right amount of thyroid hormones. But in some, this device breaks down.

1.2 THE OVERACTIVE THYROID

In a few humans, the thyroid gland can grow to be over-green because of a number of genetic, physiological or manner of lifestyles elements. This ends within the overproduction of thyroid hormones, a circumstance referred to as hyperthyroidism. An car-immune condition referred to as Grave's sickness is the maximum common reason of hyperthyroidism. Further, tumours, capsules, excessive iodine and infections also can reason an hyperactive thyroid. The scenario is quite unusual, present nice in five out of every 1000 people. The maximum not unusual signs and symptoms are fast, unusual heartbeats, fatigue, tension, advanced urge for food, excellent menstrual cycles, disturbed sleep, weight reduction, hair loss, chronic shivering, sweating, and immoderate thirst. Treatment options encompass antithyroid capsules, surgical treatment or radioactive therapy.

1.Three HYPOTHYROIDISM – THE UNDERACTIVE THYROID

When thyroid hormone tiers decrease, the brain releases TSH, signalling the thyroid to get to paintings. Yet, in a few people, the thyroid gland malfunctions, failing to deliver sufficient thyroid hormones. This effects in low ranges of thyroid hormones but immoderate ranges of TSH, a situation termed hypothyroidism.

1.Four SYMPTOMS OF AN UNDERACTIVE THYROID

Thyroid hormones are crucial for the frame to function normally. Their deficiency can purpose a large quantity of signs and signs and signs starting from lifestyles-threatening to discomforting. The maximum common symptoms consist of fatigue, weight gain, decreased urge for food and depression. However, the precise signs experienced thru the usage of an character can rely on their age, gender or race. The desk comprehensively summarises the symptoms and symptoms because of hypothyroidism at numerous some time.

AGE SYMPTOMS

INFANTS Respiratory distress, failure to benefit weight, horrible sucking potential, decreased stool frequency, reduced hobby and lethargy, umbilical hernia, dry pores and pores and skin with yellow pigmentation, swelling of the tongue, hoarse cry, stunted growth with susceptible muscle tissues, coarse facial abilities (massive bulging heads, extremely good scalp veins)

CHILDREN Stunted boom, behind schedule eruption of enamel, no longer on time losing of number one tooth, skeletal retardation, Muscle susceptible factor, learning problems, unusual and difficult stools, dry pores and pores and skin with yellow pigmentation, early sexual improvement, pre-mature remoted menstruation, milky discharges from nipples

ADOLESCENT Delayed onset of puberty, stunted increase, not on time eruption of everlasting teeth, uncommon and tough stools, Dry pores and pores and pores and skin with yellow pigmentation, milky discharge from nipples

YOUNG-MIDDLE AGE Fatigue, Weight advantage, Dry pores and pores and skin and bloodless intolerance, Slow questioning, Puffy eyes

Coarseness or lack of hair, Goitre or swelling of neck, Constipation, Hoarse voice

Muscle susceptible factor and cramps, Memory impairment, Decreased awareness, Irregular or heavy menses, Infertility, muscle pain, High ldl cholesterol, gradual coronary coronary heart price, coronary coronary coronary heart sickness, weight advantage, reduced urge for meals, melancholy, brittle nails, Swelling of the arm, arms, legs, ft and facial puffiness

ELDERLY Memory and intellectual impairment, Dementia, Anaemia, Depression, Heart failure, Coronary coronary coronary heart illness

1.Five HOW IS AN UNDERACTIVE THYROID DIAGNOSED?

Symptoms of hypothyroidism are not specific. 15 % of patients with hypothyroidism display no signs and signs and symptoms in any respect! Therefore, a biochemical test to determine circulating TSH values is the first-class conclusive method of assessment.

Generally, a healthy individual will have TSH levels ranging between zero.Four – four mU/L. However, this reference variety has been debated with the aid of way of medical doctors and scientists for many years. This is due to the reality TSH stages may be tormented by a large quantity of factors apart from an underactive thyroid, collectively with gender, age, ethnicity, weather/season, time of the day (night>morning), BMI, genetics, being pregnant and so forth. Thus, every character has a selected "regular" TSH variety, which your physician will determine primarily based completely in reality on your scientific records.

1.6 THE RISK FACTORS AND CAUSES

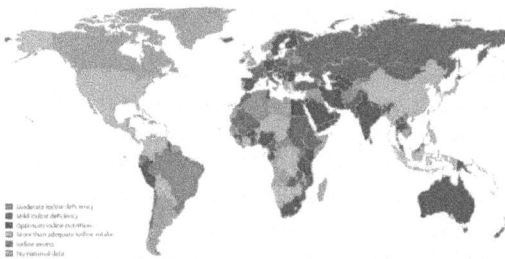

Till date, a group of genetic, lifestyle and physiological factors were related to hypothyroidism:

• IODINE DEFICIENCY is the single maximum commonplace purpose of hypothyroidism. The thyroid gland wishes iodine obtained from meals to fabricate thyroid hormones. Therefore low iodine diets can motive hypothyroidism.

Culturally, a few international locations encompass very low or very excessive iodine of their diets ensuing in immoderate expenses of hypothyroidism. This includes international places in the Middle East (Bahrain, Qatar), South

9

America (Brazil, Columbia, Venezuela, Ecuador, Chile, Guatemala, Honduras), North America (Mexico, USA), Africa (Congo, Chad, Uganda, Liberia, Namibia, Zimbabwe) and Asia (Armenia, Bhutan, Indonesia, Philippines, China).

Avoiding iodine insufficiency does now not ought to suggest growing your salt consumption. In truth, medical doctors regularly advise in competition to salt as it's far seemed to purpose high blood pressure, heart and kidney failure. Therefore, making sure the salt you operate is iodine enriched (1.Tsp >= 400mg iodine) is the pleasant and most inexpensive way to remedy this trouble.

IMAGE SOURCE: ZIMMERMAN ET AL., 2008

• HASHIMOTO'S THYROIDITIS refers to a chronic autoimmune sickness (a condition wherein the body attacks its very very own cells). The thyroid gland is regularly destroyed, ensuing in thyroid hormone deficiency. The precise cause of Hashimoto's thyroid is not appeared, but, it is idea to be due to every genetic and environmental factors.

• GENETICS is some other common threat detail for hypothyroidism. Certain human beings can be born with vehicle-immunity or mutations that burden them with a malfunctioning endocrine tool. Some toddlers are born with an underacting thyroid called congenital hypothyroidism ensuing in highbrow retardation and stunted growth (Down's syndrome, Turner's syndrome). The genetics of gender and race also can have an impact on hypothyroidism. Women, Caucasians and East - Asians are much more likely to boom an underactive thyroid.

• The presence of AUTO-IMMUNE DISEASES other than Hashimoto's also can increase the danger of developing hypothyroidism. This consists of Type 1 Diabetes, car-immune gastric atrophy, coeliac ailment, adrenal gland ailment, ovarian failure, pernicious anaemia, vitiligo and more than one sclerosis.

• Exposure to nice CHEMICALS can disrupt your thyroid. These encompass business chemical compounds (flame retardants, perchlorates), pesticides and herbicides, pollutants in patron objects (food packaging material), and heavy metals.

• AGE is appreciably associated with hypothyroidism. In older human beings, the hypothalamus, pituitary and thyroid glands undergo massive put on and tear, resulting in its malfunction.

• TREATMENT strategies which embody radioactive head and neck treatment, radioiodine remedy, bone marrow transplantation and thyroidectomy (surgical removal of all or a part of the thyroid gland) may want to have an impact at the amount of thyroid hormones.

• SMOKING influences thyroid function via a choice of factors. Chemicals in cigarettes can at once alter the cells of the thyroid gland or growth the threat of formation of nodes or tumours on this vicinity.

• HYPOTHALAMUS hypothyroidism is a exceptionally uncommon condition, due to the failure of the hypothalamus to secrete TRH (thyrotrophin- liberating hormone) ensuing in low TSH and thyroid hormone levels.

• MEDICATIONS consisting of these used to address coronary heart, psychiatric situations and most cancers might also have an effect on the ability of the thyroid gland to secrete thyroid hormones. The listing includes amiodarone, lithium, tyrosine kinase inhibitors, sunitinib, interferon-alpha, thalidomide and anti-epileptic capsules.

• It grow to be currently positioned that sufferers with BIPOLAR DISORDER have been more likely to have a malfunctioning thyroid gland, but, it isn't recognized why.

1.7 FACTORS THAT REQUIRE SPECIAL ATTENTION

Although thyroid hormone deficiency could have an effect on a number of organs inside the frame, below we summarize some elements that have to be monitored even after starting treatment for hypothyroidism.

THE HEART : Cardiovascular diseases are the place's biggest contributor to early dying. Insufficient thyroid hormones reduce coronary heart rate, increase blood strain, deposit fats internal arteries, growth ldl cholesterol and motive other dysfunctions that result in coronary heart disease. The impact of the thyroid on the coronary heart additionally may be indirect. For instance, hypothyroidism will growth metabolism, waist circumference and weight – all of that may purpose further issues on your coronary coronary heart. Patients with hypothyroidism have to take particular care in their coronary

coronary coronary heart through following a healthful food regimen and exercising time desk. Risk populations elderly over 60 must go through normal coronary heart check-usato ensure any problems may be caught early on. ?

DEPRESSION: Depression is an often-neglected ailment that reasons intense mortality, morbidity and incapacity. Hypothyroidism can bring about severe, continual depression, that persists even after thyroid remedy. Further, the drug treatments used to address thyroid are identified to intrude with drugs treating depression. Therefore, patients at immoderate chance which embody ladies and the elderly should pay unique attention to their moods. Do now not hesitate to invite for help even as crucial. If your low moods persist however thyroid remedy, your medical doctor can prescribe a big type of anti-depressants than can reduce the weight. ?

PREGNANCY: Insufficient degrees of thyroid hormones can intrude with the discharge of eggs from the ovary, resulting in infertility. In most times, infertility can be corrected with the resource of manner of really treating the underlying hypothyroidism. Further, girls are at excessive hazard of growing hypothyroidism each in the course of being pregnant and put up-partum. Although the underlying mechanism isn't virtually understood, being pregnant motives swelling and infection of the thyroid, causing it to almost double in length. Thyroid hormone deficiency in some unspecified time in the future of being pregnant may have an impact on the mother and reason severe developmental troubles within the foetus. In maximum ladies, hypothyroidism regresses surely publish-partum without any treatment. But in some persisting instances, your health practitioner may prescribe thyroid remedies. Thyroid and TSH levels need to be continuously monitored in some unspecified time in the future of being pregnant to defend each the mother and infant. ?

KIDNEY: Kidney failure or chronic kidney disease is an unfortunate associate of hypothyroidism. Kidneys want triiodothyronine to flush pollution and wastes out of your body. Therefore thyroid deficiency can cause kidney sickness, ensuing in inflamed, swollen kidneys. Patients who experience common urination, swollen ankles, fatigue, confusion, breathlessness, an?aemia, dry itchy pores and pores and skin and muscle cramps even after thyroid remedy should immediately touch a healthcare issuer for an extensive kidney take a look at-up.

1.Eight EVERYTHING YOU NEED TO KNOW ABOUT HORMONE REPLACEMENT THERAPY

Thyroid hormone deficiency if left untreated effects in crippling troubles beginning from slight signs like fatigue and weight benefit to morbid signs and symptoms and signs and symptoms and symptoms and symptoms like highbrow health troubles, coronary coronary heart sickness and coma. In pregnant girls, untreated hypothyroidism can bring about crucial harm to the foetus, inflicting starting defects, developmental and highbrow issues. Replacement remedy with thyroid hormone is the maximum generally used remedy for hypothyroidism.

1.Nine LEVOTHYROXINE

A synthetic thyroid hormone education modified into first synthetic via Dr George Murray in 1891, thru extracting sheep thyroid hormones. A decade later, animal thyroid extracts have been remoted and synthetic for oral consumption. However, animals include almost 2-3-times higher concentrations of hormones compared to human beings. Therefore, those have been not gold widespread for treatment.

In 1958, the invention of sodium salt enabled the invention of human thyroxine and triiodothyronine. Synthetic arrangements of human thyroxine, furthermore referred to as levothyroxine or L-T4 were first synthetic within the Nineteen Sixties and remains the primary drug used to treat hypothyroidism. Levothyroxine is the world's most generally used drug, with almost 104.7 million prescriptions within the US on my own.

Thyroid hormone preparations currently to be had inside the market are of sorts: herbal or synthetic. Natural desiccated thyroid arrangements are obtained from animals and can incorporate heaps better concentrations than artificial arrangements. Consult your medical doctor earlier than using any natural education to make sure thyrotoxicosis (progressed thyroid hormones within the bloodstream) does now not stand up.

Synthetic levothyroxine (supplied under brand names Levoxyl, Synthroid, Tirosint, Unithroid and so forth) gives a herbal, controlled dosage of thyroxine in assessment to herbal preparations. However, versions in attention can exist among manufacturers, consequently they need to in no way be switched with out consulting your clinical health practitioner.

Typically, hormone opportunity therapy is sustained inside the path of life, with regular blood checks to check TSH degrees. Since levothyroxine is extra with out difficulty absorbed by means of the small gut on an empty stomach, it's far counseled to take the medicine within the morning, 30-60 mins before breakfast.

1.10 HOW MUCH LEVOTHYROXINE DO YOU NEED?

The American Thyroid association describes the right each day dose of levothyroxine as 1•five–1•eight µg consistent with kg of bodyweight. However, your scientific health practitioner will decide the dosage you require primarily based to your age, BMI, gender and certainly one of a kind factors, a number of which is probably indexed under.

• The presence of related illnesses alongside aspect coronary coronary heart sickness, Type 1 diabetes, automobile-immune illnesses and so forth will have an impact on the quantity of levothyroxine you may need. For instance, patients with coronary coronary coronary heart sickness need to start with small doses that are regularly advanced to allow the coronary coronary heart to regulate to the medication.

• Pregnant women generally require better doses to recovery their malfunctioning thyroid.

• Patients with gastric problems like coeliac disorder, atrophic gastritis and so forth show off very low absorption of the medication. In such times, liquid or clean gel capsules of levothyroxine can be administered.

• Patients who have had bariatric surgical procedure furthermore display off very low absorption of levothyroxine.

• In some times, levothyroxine can have interaction with different medicinal drugs which include calcium carbonate, aluminium-containing antacids, sucralfate, iron nutritional dietary supplements, cholestyramine, sevelamer, ciprofloxacin, raloxifene, orlistat and calcium dietary supplements.

• Genetics can also have an impact on the absorption of the medication. Individuals who have mutations in genes essential for thyroid feature usually display off low absorption.

Therefore, you need to ensure to tell your health practitioner approximately your specific scientific facts.

The purpose of hormone replacement remedy is to restore normal TSH and thyroxine degrees, at the same time as reducing or stopping signs and symptoms and signs and symptoms. Yet, nearly 35% of patients treated with levothyroxine do now not benefit their goal.

Over/beneath treatment of thyroid should have important consequences on health, including insomnia, coronary heart palpitations, expanded urge for food, weight advantage, coronary heart assaults, and osteoporosis. You want to ensure you comply with your medical doctors' commands cautiously and inform them if you have forgotten or ignored taking your medicine. Annual TSH take a look at-united statesalso can assist trap any troubles with treatment, early.

1.11 NEXT GENERATION TREATMENTS

Nearly five–10% of patients who gain ordinary thyroid hormone stages keep to expose signs and symptoms and symptoms. So clinical medical doctors have all commenced out to bear in thoughts novel new strategies for treatment.

Combination restoration methods the usage of Levothyroxine and liothyronine have nowadays received reputation. Liothyronine refers back to the artificial activated shape of thyroxine. Inclusion of liothyronine circumvents the need for the body to prompt thyroxine.

Some research preserve that mixture treatment does now not fare better than levothyroxine monotherapy, with the American thyroid association going as a ways as to discourage aggregate treatments because of uncertainty regarding long term safety. However, If you're experiencing persistent debilitating signs and symptoms and signs and symptoms and symptoms, it is probably profitable to ask your health practitioner if combination treatment is proper for you.

The destiny of healthcare is custom designed treatment in which every person's genes will decide the shape of medication they're prescribed. For example, research have demonstrated sufferers with mutations within the DIO2 gene exhibit low levothyroxine absorption. Gene-based totally definitely totally treatment stays in its early stages, with only some gene remedies being accredited with the aid of regulatory bodies. Nevertheless, it is an exciting prospect to sit up straight for.

1.12 THE DO'S AND DONTS – A SUMMARY

• Don't take your medicinal drug with food: Levothyroxine need to be taken on an empty belly, one hour in advance than meals consumption.

• Don't prevent the drug whilst your signs and symptoms are resolved. The symptoms and symptoms will truly re-seem.

• Don't mixture levothyroxine with exceptional medicinal drugs along aspect nutritional supplements or antacids.

• Don't change remedy manufacturers without consulting your doctor.

• Don't devour food devices rich in soy and fibre, including papaya, coffee, grapefruits, walnuts, cotton seeds and so on, as they intervene with levothyroxine absorption.

• Do inform your medical doctor if your signs preserve to persist.

• Do inform your medical health practitioner if you have overdosed or forgotten to take your medicine.

• Do test TSH levels yearly.

• Do inform your health practitioner in case you are starting any new pills collectively with begin manipulate tablets, testosterone, melancholy medicines, oestrogen or seizure capsules.

• Do save levothyroxine capsules faraway from moderate, in dry conditions.

Chapter 2: Prevention

"Prevention is better than treatment." "A sew in time saves nine." "Better solid than sorry"

These are just some of the numerous sayings ingrained in us because of the fact we had been kids. We are constantly counseled to be careful and attempt to keep away from detrimental effects as opposed to discover a answer for them.

This applies to our fitness too. We take vaccines to prevent diseases and growth immunity toward them, so why not take a few greater steps to save you getting one-of-a-kind sicknesses for which there are not any vaccines for.

There isn't any vaccine for illnesses due to the incorrect functioning of the thyroid gland, so proper proper here are a few precautions you could take:

Consume enough iodine:

Iodine performs a crucial position inside the normal manufacturing of the thyroid hormone. It is critical which you eat the prescribed amount of iodine to prevent so that it will prevent iodine deficiency in your body. But, make certain you do no longer devour an excessive amount of iodine, as excessive iodine intake results for your body getting autoimmune thyroiditis that has comparable signs and symptoms and signs and signs and symptoms as Hashimoto's. Foods to devour: eggs, iodized salt, milk, dried sea weed, cod, shrimp, dried prunes, strawberries, bananas, yogurt and lobster.

Reduce or limit your soy product consumption:

Soy merchandise will be predisposed to suppress the natural thyroid function, resulting in hypothyroidism. A lot of women take immoderate quantities of soy products to counter the signs and symptoms and signs and symptoms of menopause, but they're at a honestly excessive chance of getting thyroid troubles. Eat complement substances to get your protein intake, in place of the soy products. Foods to devour: hen, lamb, pork, beef, lentils, beans, nuts and legumes.

Avoid taking thyroid dietary supplements

A lot of the thyroid nutritional dietary dietary supplements have sea weed or animal extracts in them and are supplied very with out trouble over-the-counter without an entire lot regulation. This results in you now not know-how how a extraordinary deal of the factors are there inside the supplements and they'll have a terrible effect for your frame. If you definitely think you want nutritional supplements, consult your physician and ask them to prescribe a few nutritional supplements for you. Do now not eat any tablets without consulting your medical doctor.

Ask for a thyroid collar:

This can be very critical. Radiation from the x ray system has a totally notable effect for your thyroid gland and in immoderate cases; it can result in thyroid most cancers. Always ask the technician for a lead collar sooner or later of an x ray of the top, dentures, neck, or collarbone area, or a mammogram to protect you from future thyroid associated problems.

Quit Smoking:

Though smoking doesn't have a direct impact for your thyroid gland, smoking can irritate some of your symptoms and your sickness at a completely short price.

Beware of fluoride:

Fluoride is commonly prescribed to hyperthyroid patients to slow down the manufacturing of the thyroid hormone. This is why; in case you eat immoderate fluoride you can gradual down your thyroid gland and suffer from hypothyroid.

Today, our water, toothpastes, dental rinses, mouth washes and maximum special dental related treatments contain fluoride. Limit your fluoride consumption thru keeping off merchandise that encompass fluoride in them.

Follow those instructions to the 'T' and be assured you may have a healthy thyroid which acquired't provide you with any troubles within the destiny.

I would like to reiterate that earlier than beginning any nutritional dietary supplements or protecting capsules please are seeking advice from your doctor; it's miles higher to ensure than consume a few component that is much more likely to motive issues later in lifestyles.

Chapter 3: Soup Recipes For Hypothyroidism

Asparagus, Fennel and Dill Soup

Serves: three-4

Ingredients:

? 5 oz... Asparagus, sliced

? 5 oz.. Fennel bulbs, chopped

? five ozsnap peas, stringed, chopped

? 1 small bunch green onions, chopped

? ¾ teaspoon sea salt or to taste

? 1 large leek

? 1 ½ - 2 tablespoons lemon juice or to taste

? Freshly ground pepper to flavor

? 2 cups water

? 1 ½ tablespoons brown rice

? 1 tablespoon olive oil

? ¼ cup sparkling mint leaves

? ¼ cup glowing dill

? 1 ½ cups vegetable broth or chicken broth

? Zest of 1 lemon

? Garnish with fruity inexperienced olive oil

Method:

1. Place the asparagus, snap peas and fennel bulbs in a soup pot. Add water.

2. Place the pot over medium warmth. Bring to the boil. Add salt and rice to it.

three. Lower warm temperature and cover with a lid. Simmer for about 20-25 mins.

four. Meanwhile, region a small pan over medium warmth. Add oil. When the oil is heated, upload the inexperienced onions, sauté for a few minutes.

five. Add a pinch of salt. Sauté until golden brown. Transfer into the soup pot.

6. Add dill, mint and the vegetable broth to the pot. Simmer for some extra mins. Turn off the warmth. Cool for awhile.

7. Transfer right into a blender and mix till clean. Pour it decrease again into the pot.

8. Place the pot over medium low warmness. Simmer again. Add pepper powder and lemon juice. Taste and regulate the seasoning and lemon juice if essential.

9. Pour the soup into soup bowls and positioned a few drops of fruity green olive oil and serve warm.

Meatball Soup

Serves: eight

?   21 oz. Minced or ground beef or beef or a mixture of each

?   2 medium carrots, thinly sliced

?   2 cups cabbage, finely chopped

?   2 medium onions, finely chopped

? 1 ½ cups iciness squash or courgette, reduce into small cubes

? 3 tablespoons garlic, chopped

? four-5 tablespoons home made sauerkraut

? Salt to taste

? Cayenne pepper to taste

? Fresh dill, finely chopped to garnish

? Yogurt to garnish

Method:

1. Add floor meat proper into a bowl. Make small balls of the combination of about ¾ inch diameter.

2. Place a soup pot over medium warmth. Add approximately 8-10 cups water. Bring to the boil.

3. Add salt and cayenne pepper and stir.

4. Drop the meatballs in the water. Drop one by one.

5. Lower warmth to low. Cover with a lid. Simmer for round half-hour.

6. Add carrot, cabbage, onions and wintry climate squash.

7. Cover the lid and simmer till greens are easy.

8. Add garlic and stir. Turn off warmth. Let it cowl and sit down for some time.

nine. Add sauerkraut and stir.

10. Ladle into soup bowls and serve garnished with dill and yogurt.

Lentil Stew

Serves: 8

Ingredients:

? 2 pounds brown lentils, rinsed, soaked in water for 1-5 hours

? 8 medium sticks celery, chopped

? 2 bay leaves

? 2 big yellow onions, chopped

? eight cloves garlic, chopped

? 6 teaspoons sea salt or to flavor

? Freshly ground pepper to flavor

? 1 1/three cups sparkling cilantro, chopped

? 8 huge carrots, chopped

? 6 small yellow potatoes

? 4 teaspoons easy thyme, chopped or 8 teaspoons dried thyme

? eight tablespoons olive oil

? 4 teaspoons cumin seeds, roasted, floor

? Juice of a lemon

? 4 cups hen stock or vegetable inventory

? 2 cups parsley, chopped

Method:

1. Add lentils proper right into a soup pot. Pour approximately 15 cups water, bay leaf, carrots, celery and sweet potatoes into it.

2. Place the pot over medium warmth. Bring to the boil.

3. Lower warm temperature and simmer till veggies and lentils are soft. It need to take as a minimum an hour.

four. Meanwhile, region a skillet over medium warmth. Add oil. When the oil is heated, upload garlic and onion and sauté till translucent. Transfer into the soup. Stir and permit it keep simmering until mild.

five. During the closing 15 minutes of cooking, add inventory, cumin, salt and lemon juice.

6. Remove from warm temperature. Add cilantro, parsley, salt and pepper. Stir

7. Ladle into soup bowls and serve.

Mushroom Soup

Serves: 6

Ingredients:

? 2 medium onions, finely chopped

? 2 tablespoons sunflower oil

? 2.2 pounds mushrooms, finely chopped

? 2 gluten free vegetable stock cubes

? Salt to taste

? Pepper to flavor

? Handful smooth parsley, chopped

? 6 teaspoons corn flour combined with 2 tablespoons water

? 1 cup unmarried cream

Method:

1. Place a huge soup pot over medium warmness. Add oil. When the oil is heated, upload onions and sauté until golden brown.

2. Stir inside the mushrooms and cook dinner dinner for 4-5 mins. Stir continuously.

3. Boil 5 cups water and add stock cubes into it. Let it dissolve.

4. Pour inventory into the soup pot. Add parsley, salt and pepper and bring to the boil.

5. Lower warmth and cover with a lid. Simmer for 15-20 minutes.

6. Add corn flour combination and stir continuously till thick.

7. Add cream and stir.

8. Ladle into soup bowls and serve.

Chapter 4: Thyroid Nourishing Foods

Nutrition is ready consuming a healthy balanced diet plan essential for fitness and boom? It is important to be aware that dietary health is described due to the fact the era that interprets the vitamins and exclusive meals substances to preserve fitness, increase, and replica within the frame and prevent disease? Nutrition includes and impacts ingestion, absorption, biosynthesis, catabolism, and excretion of the body's system? Therefore, we literal y are what we eat! Listed under are the have to-have proteins, minerals, and nutrients and meals required for thyroid and bodily fitness?

Healthy Proteins:

•

Require nicely digestion for absorption

•

Poultry

-

Fish and seafood

-

Thyrosine: an amino acid positioned in proteins that allows make thyroid hormones

sixteen

 The Guide to Natural Thyroid Healing Iron:

-

Needed for superior thyroid characteristic

-

Supports T4 to T3 conversion

-

Vegetarian

-

Green leafy greens

-

Beans

-

Peas

-

Dried raisins and apricots

-

Quinoa

-

Animal

-

Poultry

-

Vegetarian belongings are extra tough to digest Zinc:

-

Immune nutrient that helps T4 to T3 conversion

-

Animal food

- Seafood

- Plant deliver

- Pumpkin seeds

- Chickpeas

Vitamin A:

- Immune nutrient wanted for T4 to T3 conversion

- Organ meats: especial y liver

- Egg yolks: complete herbal free range eggs

-

Common deficiency in hypothyroid individuals and diabetics

17

 Dr. Kristina Ray Iodine:

- Seaweed

- Seafood: especial y shrimp and crab

- Do not supplement without labs and addressing selenium first

Selenium:

- Common deficiency due to soil

- Brazil nuts eight–9 a day

- Supplement hundred mcg an afternoon

-

Critical nutrient for T4 synthesis and T4 to T3

conversion

Antioxidants:

-

Fights off irritation

-

Berries

-

Coniferous greens

Magnesium

-

Helps with T4 to T3 conversion

-

Helps to make T4

-

Needed for the absorption of vitamins
Probiotics

•

S? Boulardi, L? Plantarum, L? Rhamnosus
(talk with health practitioner earlier to
apply)

•

May be beneficial to calm the immune
system

•

Decreases intestine inflammation

18

The Guide to Natural Thyroid Healing
Fruits and veggies are important to growth
antioxidants, decrease oxidative strain and
reduce infection?

Berries and cruciferous veggies are KEY!

Cruciferous greens encompass:

•

cauliflower

•

cabbage, kale

•

garden cress

•

bok choy

•

broccoli

•

Brussels sprouts

•

and comparable inexperienced leafy vegetables Fruits and veggies are loaded with nutrients that fight viruses, micro organism, pathogens, and help the immune machine? They provide important vitamins wanted for a wholesome body and thyroid?

Other essential elements, herbs and dietary dietary supplements:

-

Morning celery water: A natural cleanser that aids within the breakdown of food and allows the liver and manufacturing of the thyroid hormone?

-

Cilantro: Helps flush pollution like heavy metals and viruses?

-

Wild blueberries: High in antioxidants that assist to repair and keep thyroid tissue? They additionally help to eliminate heavy metallic pollutants?

19

Dr. Kristina Ray

-

Thyme: Mega antiviral that knocks down viral load?

-

Licorice: Powerful herb that restores adrenals, permits the kidneys and lowers contamination?

- Turmeric: Anti-inflammatory, decreases viral load and enables restore the thyroid?

-

Sprouts: High in zinc and selenium and boosts the immune tool and includes micronutrients that nourish the thyroid?

- Basil: Antiviral houses?

-

Magnesium: Many health benefits vital for the frame?

-

Omega 3s (salmon): Decreases infection inside the body?

-

Vitamin C: Strengthens the complete immune device?

-

Vitamin D: Immune nutrient? Helps with the absorption of vitamins?

-

Ginger: Powerful antiviral?

-

Garlic: Antiviral and antibacterial?

-

Lemons and limes: Improve digestion, balance sodium and activate electrolytes?

-

Onion: Potent antiviral and helps the immune device?

20

The Guide to Natural Thyroid Healing

-

Raw honey: Antiviral, antibacterial, and the glucose feeds the thyroid gland?

-

Spirulina: An alga this is an antiviral, receives rid of heavy metals and boosts the immune device?

-

Cats Claw: Destroys viruses and bacteria that bring about inflammation

-

Elderberry: Strengthens the immune gadget?

Let's now not neglect about about the significance of REST, SLEEP and PLAY! Long-term pressure will save you the thyroid from running properly?

While on the thyroid recovery adventure, it may be encouraged thru your healthcare practitioner to take a thyroid complement and slowly decrease the dose till your thyroid starts offevolved offevolved working proficiently on its non-public? If desired, the most commonplace thyroid medicinal tablets are synthetic pharmaceutical capsules called: Synthroid, levothyroxine, Levoxyl, Levothroid, Thyrolar, and liotrix? These pills mimic T4 and do no longer provide T3

assist? A natural thyroid remedy gives T4 and T3 help and is more recognizable to the body considering it's far herbal? The preference is yours? I personal y switched from Synthroid to a herbal thyroid medicine and felt plenty higher? It end up no marvel that my body responded higher to a herbal supplement providing each vital 21

Dr. Kristina Ray thyroid hormones? Consult collectively with your medical doctor regarding the remarkable thyroid treatment manipulate for you?

Natural thyroid medicinal drugs consist of:

-

Armour thyroid (maximum common)

-

Nature thyroid

The thyroid is a complicated organ and to properly heal you need to make sure you take the ideal steps within the proper order with an remarkable healthcare team for most eye-catching recuperation? If you have got have been given a couple of autoimmune troubles or more than one health issues, your recuperation machine can also require hobby to the place of maximum significance and your thyroid may take longer to get higher? Each individual's recuperation adventure is specific? Taking steps within the course of a greater in shape way of life will useful resource the restoration of your frame?

I can't pressure sufficient the significance of speakme alongside facet your medical doctor and allied healthcare practitioners to installation a recreation plan that is good for you and your recuperation?

Chapter 5: An Ideal Thyroid Diet

The thyroid calls for unique minerals or nutrients for optimum functionality. Research studies have set up that even though everybody has a selected nutrient requirement, a few key vitamins are crucial for without a doubt every person. These vitamins encompass:

Iodine

This hint detail has been placed to be the maximum essential in keeping perfect popular usual performance of thyroid hormone. This is because of the fact your frame calls for the essential building blocks provided via iodine in making sure proper functioning of numerous body metabolisms. Out of those hormones, T3 and T4 are the most crucial and iodine-preserving hormones the frame desires.

Primary belongings of iodine encompass iodized sea salt, sea veggies collectively with kelp, arame and Kombu, in addition to sea meals collectively with salmon, shrimp, oysters, clams and haddock. You also can achieve iodine from secondary assets consisting of lima beans, mushrooms, asparagus, garlic, spinach, summer season squash and eggs.

Selenium

This hint element consists of enzymes that coat the thyroid gland from consequences of strain, therefore running as a "detox". The cleansing way guarantees your frame can excrete chemical and oxidative stress, which interferes with the everyday functioning of the frame. Taking selenium-primarily based proteins is critical in tracking the synthesis of hormones, therefore changing T4 hormone to the maximum utilizable form of T3.

The proteins mixed with enzymes can artwork efficiently in monitoring the metabolic way, to ensure pleasant the maximum appropriate quantities of thyroid quantities are furnished. Selenium is also very critical in tracking and ensuring endured supply of iodine in your frame.

Selenium is obviously positioned in plants together with soybeans, mushrooms, sunflower seeds and Brazil nuts and animals like tuna, organ meats and red meat.

Trace Metals

You need 3 trace metals for your vitamins comprising of copper, zinc and iron to enhance the functioning of thyroid stimulating hormone. Research has set up that having every a hyperactive and underactive thyroid can reason deficiencies of zinc that reduce the quantity of thyroid hormone. A low degree of iron is also chargeable for decreased interest of thyroid, which whilst combined with iodine deficiency, calls for iron to repair thyroid imbalance.

On the opposite hand, you want copper to improve the producing of thyroid stimulating hormone and T4 hormone; copper deficiency has been attributed to causing coronary coronary heart troubles and immoderate cholesterols in people with thyroid issues. You want T4 hormone in regulation of ldl cholesterol to your frame.

You can acquire zinc from soybeans, walnuts, complete grains, almonds, turkey, lamb, ginger root, sardines, cauliflower, maple syrup and sparkling oysters. Copper is decided in pork, nuts, beans, tomato paste, dark chocolate, lobster, sunflower seeds, and crabmeat. Iron is located in oysters, lentils, pumpkin seeds, organ meats, clams and blackstrap molasses.

Antioxidants and nutrients

Antioxidants are very critical in coping with degenerative ailments and enhance the developing older approach. You moreover need vitamins along with beta-carotene also referred to as Vitamin A, vitamins C and E to assist the thyroid gland to oxidize ongoing strain. You may additionally additionally have lethal tiers of oxidative strain if you are affected by the Graves illness, a common state of affairs of hyperactive thyroid.

Beta-carotene is determined in carrots, candy potatoes, lettuce, broccoli, and wintry weather squash. You can advantage vitamins C from papaya, citrus, Brussels sprouts, parsley, peppers, and straw berries. You can gather diet E from liver, peanuts, asparagus, almonds, and leafy inexperienced veggies.

Having a hyperactive thyroid calls for ok oxygen deliver, in which in lengthy-time period, the supply of oxygen effects into pilling up of oxygenated compounds which is probably poisonous to body cells. Your medical health practitioner can also recommendation that you take antioxidants to restrict oxidative stress outcomes. Taking the ones antioxidants together with B nutrients like Vitamin B2,

B3 and B6 is normally endorsed. Egg yolks and mushrooms are wealthy sources of vitamins B2 whilst chicken and rice bran includes diet B3, which is also referred to as niacin. To achieve vitamin B6, eating sea fish, brown rice, bananas, and brewer's yeast can offer your body with the nutrients B6 it dreams.

Chapter 6: 7 Step Plan

Below are 7 Steps you can take to restructure your lifestyles so that you can reduce the signs and symptoms and symptoms and symptoms of your thyroid.

Step 1: Take Stock of your state of affairs. Analysis your way of existence, what you are consuming, workout, artwork situation, your environment and make notes of all devices which can make a contribution to your thyroid

For this you'll need a pocket book and write down your each day sports activities sports and eating habits for one week so you can assessment it.

Step 2: Remove Toxin. Cut out sugar, or update it for weight loss plan for the instant till you may reduce out sugar altogether. This method no clean liquids, biscuits, desserts, cookies or desserts. Eat prevent result instead. Cut out flavored yogurts as they encompass excessive degrees of sugar. Cut out snacking on afternoon chocolate and replace it with something savory.

Cut out Caffeine; So no Coke, No Strong Tea, No Coffee. Go Decafe for teas and coffees.

Remove Food Allergies; if you are allergic to a few aspect prevent ingesting it.

Remove Goitrous Food – If you be afflicted by hypothyroidism Goiter is a substance that slows down the thyroid. It is decided in bok choy, broccoli, Brussels' sprouts, cabbage, cauliflower, kale, mustard greens, radishes, soy, soy milk, soy lecithin (frequently used as filler in vegetarian food) and tofu. Cooking them reduces their goitrous houses but you have to though restriction them inside the elimination section

Step 3: Healing your Thyroid.

- usually natural, they'll be greater nutrients-packed and free of hormones which may be identified to interrupting our endocrine tool

- meat ought to be at the least organic however pasture-raised is exquisite. We need to remove antibiotics and increase hormones from our eating regimen

- food that is FERMENTED the conventional way, so things like sauerkraut, kimchi, kefir, domestic made yoghurt, kombucha tea are all rich in probiotics.

Add PROTEINS and FATS

They are the building blocks of your digestive song and our hormones. We are fats-o-phobic in America and low-fat diets are one of the worse matters that we invented. Europeans and Asians have fat-rich diets (historically) and enjoy an lousy lot higher health than we do. Good fats hints: avocados, walnuts, coconut oil, coconut butter. Animal fats are the amazing in restoring a digestion; ghee (clarified butter), butter, chook and beef fats are crucial but need to be rendered and not in fried/processed shape.

Add PROBIOTICS are key in restoring your digestive song

Everyone has bacteria in their digestive tract, or gut, that is crucial to the characteristic of the human frame. A healthful adult has approximately 1.Five – 2 kg of micro organism in their gut, each pinnacle and horrible. Normal degrees of micro organism, or plant life, inside the gut protects in opposition to invaders, undigested meals, pollution, and parasites. When the high-quality and terrible bacteria inside the intestine get out of whack (i.E. Extra bad than correct), a whole host of horrible reactions can get up within the body. Undigested meals can leak via into the bloodstream causing meals allergies and intolerances, vitamins and minerals to not be absorbed, leading to deficiency, the lousy micro organism to provide a whole host of pollution, and the immune tool to no longer characteristic properly.

Here are examples of traditionally fermented meals you may include to your eating regimen:

Sauerkraut (pick out properly fermented, now not in vinegar)

Kim chee (Korean fermented greens)

Yoghurt (that is my recipe to make your non-public yoghurt)

Kefir (has one among a type bacteria than yoghurt, moreover first-rate beneficial)

Kombucha tea

Vegetable medley (fermented)

Coconut water kefir

Step four: Supplement your Diet with Supplements to reinforce your Body

Below are 5 nutritional dietary supplements you can keep in mind taking for best Thyroid fitness.

1. Iodine. Iodine is critical for the formation of the thyroid hormones. Because of this, many healthcare experts expect that people with a hyperthyroid circumstance have a further of iodine, which commonly isn't the case. For people with Hashimoto's Thyroiditis, they need to not take iodine till the autoimmune response is addressed. While many humans with this case are iodine negative, their signs and signs and symptoms and signs will commonly get worse in the occasion that they take iodine in advance than addressing the immune gadget trouble.

Your pharmacy or doctor have to in a function that will help you with Iodine dosage

2. Vitamin D. Vitamin D is surprisingly vital in immunity, and because of this can be

very vital for helping people with autoimmune thyroid disorders, inclusive of Graves' Disease and Hashimoto's Thyroiditis. But even in humans with "normal" thyroid conditions, it's miles clever to discover if you are weight loss program D deficient, that might with out problem be decided through a simple blood take a look at.

Like supplementing with iodine, taking Vitamin D dietary supplements is specifically a lot less pricey, and might do wonders for your fitness. Of route a massive deliver of Vitamin D is the solar, so on the identical time as taking supplements can assist, you furthermore may need to attempt to get a few each day sun exposure as nicely.

3. Selenium. In order for T4 to get transformed to T3, an enzyme that includes selenium is crucial. As a give up end result, a deficiency in selenium will have an effect in this conversion approach,

and as a end result impair thyroid function. The outstanding records is that most human beings can gain all of the selenium they need thru eating one or raw Brazil nuts every day. If you don't like Brazil nuts then garlic is likewise a fantastic deliver of selenium.

four. Magnesium. Magnesium is an essential mineral to take, as many humans are magnesium deficient. In addition to getting magnesium from your weight loss program through leafy green greens, whole grains, and top notch property, one need to additionally do not forget taking a magnesium complement. This is even greater essential in case you are supplementing with iodine, as magnesium is vital for the right absorption of iodine.

five. B Vitamins. Taking B Vitamins is likewise important for most beneficial thyroid health. Like magnesium, taking B nutrients is crucial for really absolutely everyone supplementing with iodine. The motive for that is because of the truth the B Vitamins (specifically B2 and B3) assist with the usage of iodine at the mobile stage. But even for those human beings with a thyroid situation who aren't iodine poor, it but is a splendid concept to take B nutrients on a each day foundation. B nutrients furthermore help you to soak up Vitamin D

Consult our pharmacy or doctor or naturopathy for an superb selection of high grade dietary supplements.

Step five: Exercise and Relax and Rest and Let your body Heal

This is probable the toughest to alternate. We all live in a very busy worldwide so locating time to loosen up is tough. The fantastic way to do is to replace some easy every day sports with exercise so giving your self an additional 30minutes a day will help to decorate your immunity in order to help to regular your thyroid. You could in all likelihood even discover that walking an additional 10minutes to paintings or to a genuinely one in all a type café makes you feel greater cushty.

Find time to rest so your body will heal. They say that the super natural healer inside the global is sleep because it permits your frame to heal itself the way it is supposed to be. So if you may locate time to rest your head on your table on the place of job for a arvo nap of 15-20minutes then do it. Otherwise, hold in mind taking a nap whilst you get domestic around 6pm in advance than dinner. You would likely revel in hungry however you is probably greater tired than hungry. Try to have a lie down and decrease out the world for 30minutes in advance than cooking dinner and this could paintings to loosen up and heal your frame.

I recognize you're busy however you NEED to discover time for this so you gets better and experience better

Step 6: Heat Therapy and Relaxation

Try a sauna or Infra-red remedy or mild remedy. They say that one hour of infra-crimson treatment is equivalent to two hours at the gym and you begin to sweat out your pollutants. The infra-purple blankets are cheaper to shop for off ebay so that you can keep in mind having them at domestic that will help you detox. They are the contemporary-day day in recovery and toxin elimination. They will assist you to constantly maintain your body nicely circulated and at the equal time dispose of pollutants. You will discover it most fun and that allows you to moreover assist your body heal.

Step 7: Meditation and Giving it time

I don't need to sound like a new age guru however if you surely spend some time far from the stresses of your life then you'll be capable of reduce the pollution in your body. Stress is the number one purpose for an entire lot of chronic infection within the intervening time because of the truth the Stress hormones launch pollution into your body. This is why such numerous human beings advocate mediation. If you may't meditate then don't fear. The maximum crucial trouble is as quick as a day to give your self a time that you spend attention on healing yourself so recall restoration and be exquisite and remind your frame that that is the point of interest and the most essential factor to you inside the within the period in-between. In life you could simplest remedy what you cognizance on so spend actually 10-15 mins an afternoon inside the morning in advance than paintings and interest on the outstanding and interest on recuperation your frame after which be affected person and deliver your frame time to heal.

Chapter 7: Other Thyroid-Related Dysfunctions

An enlarged thyroid gland is referred to as a goitre. The thyroid gland is positioned within the the front of the windpipe. It produces and secretes hormones that modify increase and metabolism. Mostly the stated instances are categorized as easy goitres due to the fact they do no longer contain any contamination or any detriment to thyroid characteristic, no seen signs and symptoms and signs and often having no obvious motive.

The severity of the symptoms and signs and symptoms var regarding an person. Most of the goitres produce no outstanding signs and symptoms and signs and symptoms, however at the same time as the symptoms and signs and signs and symptoms and signs arise, someone feels tightness, cough, and hoarseness, hassle in swallowing or in intense instances, trouble respiration with a immoderate pitch sound.

The signs of an overactive thyroid can cause signs and symptoms and symptoms like anxiety, palpitations, hyperactivity, accelerated sweating, heat allergic reaction, fatigue, extended urge for food, lack of hair and weight reduction. The signs and symptoms of an underactive thyroid can reason signs and symptoms like cold intolerance, constipation, forgetfulness, person adjustments, hair loss, and weight gain.

14.1.1 Various Causes of Goitre

Different situations contribute to causing a goitre.

Iodine deficiency

Iodine deficiency is considered one of the essential reasons of goitre around the arena, but this is rarely a cause in countries which might be nicely-superior and wherein iodine is delivered to salt in every day everyday.

In some components of the sector, the frequency of goitre instances is stated as immoderate as 80%, i.E. In the remote mountainous regions of southeast Asia, Latin America and imperative Africa. In those cited places, the each day consumption of iodine can fall under 25 micrograms (mcg) steady with day and the infants are often born with hypothyroidism.

To adjust metabolism, the thyroid gland requires iodine to manufacture thyroid hormones.

Autoimmune illness

The important motive of goitre in developed worldwide places is an autoimmune sickness. Women which are probably over the age of 40 are at a extra hazard of goitre, especially the human beings having a own family information of this situation.

Hypothyroidism is a outcome of an underactive thyroid gland and this produces goitre. As the gland produces too little thyroid hormone, it's miles brought about to supply extra, which ends up in the swelling. Usually, that is a result of Hashimoto's thyroiditis, it's a situation in which tissues of a frame are attacked with the aid of way of manner of the frame's immune system that motives irritation of the thyroid gland.

Hyperthyroidism is a end result of an overactive thyroid gland that reasons goitre. In this example, an excessive amount of thyroid hormone is produced. Usually, this is a cease end result of Graves' Disease, an autoimmune disease wherein the body's immune gadget activates itself and assaults the thyroid gland, which reasons it to swell.

Less common reasons

Some of the masses lots much less not unusual reasons of goitre include:

Smoking ?

A chemical thiocyanate placed in tobacco smoke impacts the absorption of iodine in a frame, resulting in goitre.

Hormonal modifications ?

Menopause, being pregnant, and puberty could have an impact on thyroid function, which leads to goitre.

Thyroiditis ?

Inflammation that is due to infection of bacteria or viruses can purpose goitre.

Lithium ?

Psychiatric capsules that contain lithium can intrude with the functioning of the thyroid.

Overconsumption of iodine ?

If iodine is fed on in a big amount, then an excessive amount of iodine can also purpose goitre.

Radiation remedy ?

This can prompt a swollen thyroid, specially at the identical time as administered to the neck.

14.1.2 Diagnosis of Goiter

Goitre can satisfactory be diagnosed with a physical exam of the neck, feeling for a swelling. To test for goitre, the medical doctor also can ask the affected person to swallow. Once the health practitioner diagnoses a affected person for goitre, the underlying problems with the thyroid characteristic must be evaluated and the affected man or woman should be screened for hyperthyroidism or hypothyroidism.

TSH and T4 levels are measured in the blood to test thyroid function. A carefully managed remarks mechanism technique that TSH encourages the thyroid for the producing of greater thyroxine than is needed, even as T4 tells the thyroid to prevent generating more thyroxine.

In an overactive thyroid, TSH levels are discovered to be low or non-existent, at the identical time as T4 ranges are excessive. In people having an underactive thyroid, the alternative is actual. TSH tiers are immoderate and T4 levels are low. Triiodothyronine is every specific hormone this is measured in a few times of an overactive gland, collectively with suspected Graves' Disease.

In few instances of goitre, professional checks may be organized, i.E. Radioactive iodine test wherein a entire picture of the gland is supplied, found through an injection of radioactive iodine. Ultrasound Scan evaluates the gland and size of the goitre, and Fine-Needle Aspiration is a form of biopsy is completed to take a pattern of the cells from the gland if maximum cancers is suspected.

In goitres which might be due to overactive thyroid or hyperthyroidism, the treatment reputation is to counter the producing of greater hormone. For this reason, anti-thyroid drugs, collectively with ethionamide tablets, are given to reduce the immoderate hormone degrees progressively.

Radioactive iodine is also a treatment to lower thyroid function and to forestall hormone production that reasons hyperthyroidism.

In goitres which can be attributable to underactive thyroid or hypothyroidism, the treatment is a synthetic opportunity of thyroid hormone. The dosage of artificial thyroxine T4 is multiplied often till the frame restores the ordinary thyroid levels.

14.1.Three Goitre Surgery

Goitre surgical treatment is needed in such vital times wherein goitre is inflicting a few troubles in swallowing and problem in breathing. This surgical treatment is completed below well-known anaesthesia to dispose of a part of the thyroid gland.

14.1. Four Best Diet for Goitre

Iodine is not found in a excellent quantity in vegetation, and vegetarian food also can lack sufficient iodine. Dietary iodine is located in seafood (salmon, tuna, halibut, shrimp, and so forth.), flowers which may be grown in iodine-wealthy soil, cow's milk, and eggs (right iodine and selenium are present within the yolk).

Mostly the simple form of goitres may be avoided thru using taking a right quantity of iodine, it's far added to desk salt in many countries. A massive range of iodine nutritional supplements is likewise to be had on line. In times wherein signs and signs and symptoms are visible, energetic treatment of goitre is completed. But if the goitre is small and thyroid is functioning typically, treatment is in the critical not supplied.

14.2 Thyroid Nodules

Nodules are termed as "stable or lump having fluid" within the thyroid gland. This may additionally variety in period and area. The majority of the nodules do now not purpose any symptoms and signs and symptoms and signs and might fine be recognized at some stage in a manual examination of the thyroid gland or with the resource of doing an ultrasound of a thyroid.

Large-sized nodules may additionally bring about a seen swelling of the thyroid or neck. These nodules might also additionally reason pain, problem in swallowing and respiratory. There also are sorts of nodules that produce thyroid hormones which result in hyperthyroidism.

Around 50% of adults in America are identified with thyroid nodules. Women undergo 3 instances more than men. About 30% of girls after they attain the age of the 30s are identified with as a minimum one, on the equal time as maximum of girls boom a thyroid nodulein their50s.

14.2.1 Symptoms of Nodules

The signs and symptoms of thyroid nodules aren't masses observable. One can best look at them in a form of lump acting at the neck or a medical doctor would possibly discover those nodules in the route of a bodily examination or while CT scans or imaging exams like ultrasounds are finished for exceptional motives.

Luckily, most of the nodules display signs and symptoms and signs and signs and symptoms, but those symptoms and symptoms are manifested no longer regularly, i.E. A suffered man or woman also can revel in ache in neck, ear or jaw. One can also experience a trouble at the same time as respiration, swallowing or a tickle within the throat, if the nodule is large;hoarseness if the nodules have an impact at the nerve that controls the vocal cords. This additionally can be related to thyroid cancer. The excessive amount of thyroxine production generates a symptom of hyperthyroidism that consists of tremors, tension, unexplained weight reduction, and erratic heartbeat.

If the thyroid test effects of someone aren't in a regular range, then a person must get himself tested for nodules.

14.2.2 Causes of Nodules Formation

People stricken by Hashimoto's have nodules which may be considered to be the idea motive of thyroid nodules. Some distinct causes of thyroid nodules are given underneath:

Chronic Inflammation of the Thyroid ?

A continual infection this is connected with autoimmune thyroid conditions can also growth the chance for thyroid nodules and consequently the infection related with autoimmune thyroiditis can in addition increase nodules. With Hashimoto's, the body creates such antibodies that normal proteins produced by the usage of the thyroid gland which in flip effects within the improvement of malignant nodules that might be cancerous. This thyroid might also form pseudo-nodules which could come and move.

Nutritional deficiencies ?

Various dietary deficiencies because of loss of proper weight loss program can result in the insufficiency of iodine, selenium and Vitamin D within the frame. The deficiency of iodine in a body typically consequences in a multinodular goitre, but with Hashimoto's, the extra in iodine is a protracted manner much more likely to purpose nodules. A deficiency in selenium is likewise a capability cause of nodules and nutritional nutritional supplements used can decorate thyroid and small duration modules. Adding fish, nuts, yogurt, and fruits to our weight loss program can beautify the severity of thyroid nodules.

Toxins ?

Various pollution that enter our frame from the environment and meals can negatively have an effect on the thyroid. Most of the time this motive of nodules is disregarded. People dwelling near petrochemical enterprise regions are exposed to radiation exposure, like Chernobyl and nickel toxicity, considerably contributes to the improvement of nodules in people who be bothered with the aid of Hashimoto's disorder.

Pregnancy and Hormonal adjustments ?

Most of the time, ladies increase thyroid nodules inside the direction of pregnancy. But the purpose of nodules all through being pregnant remains no longer clean and plenty of studies advise that this may be due to negative iodine balance related with pregnancy.

H. Pylori Infections ?

H. Pylori infections are considered as a cause of Hashimoto's and a check suggests that someone stricken by Hashimoto's has been placed in almost 50% of sufferers. According to a principle of molecular mimicry, the thyroid gland is attacked with the resource of its immune device at the same time as it receives inflamed with any pathogenic organism. Such an contamination will increase the autoimmune attack at the thyroid that consequences within the manufacturing of a thyroid nodule.

Food and Diet ?

Food sensitivities are also one of the reasons for nodules as some meals assault the thyroid and increase the volume of chronic contamination. Moreover, an imbalance in blood sugars also can make a contribution to a greater risk of thyroid nodules. Overuse of fast meals and processed meals can increase the hazard of growing thyroid nodules.

 Treatment ?

Most docs endorse bodily tracking through regular checkups. Thyroid hormone suppression therapy can decrease the manufacturing of TSH and reduce the boom of thyroid tissues. Surgery can also be endorsed if the benign nodule is huge and creates problem in respiration or swallowing.

14.2.Three Diet and Lifestyle Changes to Reduce Nodules

Changes in weight loss program and manner of lifestyles patterns make a contribution hundreds to lessen thyroid nodules. Some hints are mentioned beneath:

 Add vitamins like Iodine, Selenium and Vitamin D inside the diet ?

People having low iodine stages can also gain by means of manner of using taking multivitamins with iodine like Nutrient 950 from Pure Encapsulations. People suffering from Hashimoto's want a dose of as a great deal as 250mcg of iodine regular with day that is placed to be beneficial. However, a dose above 300mcg may be inflammatory. Taking Vitamin D and Selenium dietary supplements may additionally moreover assist in the discount of thyroid nodules.

Remove pollutants from the frame ?

By assisting liver cleansing, strategies for opting non-toxic, natural personal products can help hundreds to lessen the body's toxic burden and improving top-rated thyroid health. Various fruits and veggies, together with avocadoes, apples, citrus, asparagus, green leafy veggies, beetroot and carrots are outstanding detox sellers and may be used to take away unwanted pollution from the frame and guard the thyroid and different factors of the frame.

Address underlying infections ?

Infections like H. Pylori and Blastocystis hominis are taken into consideration as a root purpose and set off Hashimoto's and expand thyroid nodules. By addressing such infections you could take away thyroid nodules further to the danger of an autoimmune attack at the thyroid. Taking vitamins E nutritional supplements and omega three oils can help enhance the immune device and can aid in doing away with any underlying infections.

Alter healthy eating plan and get rid of food sensitivities ?

Balancing blood sugar will assist masses in shrinking thyroid nodules. Also, removing common food sensitivities, like gluten and dairy, can assist in decreasing the dimensions of nodules.

Add smart dietary supplements ?

Some studies display that the removal of nodules is feasible via ingesting the systemic enzyme Wobenzym and others with turmeric. Turmeric is a effective anti-inflammatory spice and might help reduce irritation inside the thyroid gland.

Address estrogen dominance ?

Excess portions of estrogen in a body turns on the thyroid nodules. Estrogen tiers can also increase in the path of pregnancy or through the usage of shipping control drugs, but it rebalances on its very own after transport or stops the usage of medicine. However if estrogen degrees do now not rebalance even after transport or stopped the use of drugs, then one want to endure in mind specific reasons like food alteration, nutritional dietary dietary supplements, and progesterone to balance the hormones.

Give perception to Echo treatment (HIFU ablation) ?

Studies advise that a unmarried sitting of high-depth targeted ultrasound (HIFU) ablation can be greater useful than thyroidectomy. In one take a look at, it modified into determined that the patients who underwent HIFU ablation did not scar had a restrained medical institution stay and have been a good deal less probably to have voice pitch problems after a month of remedy. But this technique is handiest available currently in a few clinics in Europe.

Chapter 8: Magnesium Therapy:

It is not any mystery these days that Magnesium is vital for our fitness, healing and durability. So lots humans are depleted of this important mineral because of our current international stressors. With over 3 hundred identified skills for it in our bodies we should take top notch care to build up enough magnesium and restore our ranges. There are numerous books that have been written in this. Check out Dr. Carolyn Dean's ebook, The Magnesium Miracle or Dr. Sircus' ebook, Transdermal Magnesium Therapy. Read the ones and redecorate your health with simply this mineral by myself. These books pass into great depths to provide an reason of the way vital this mineral is. It up-regulates the immune tool, protects the cells from heavy metallic publicity, will growth brain feature, and permits osteoporosis. Contrary to famous belief, getting more calcium is often now not essential, it's miles the magnesium detail this is required to stress the calcium into the right locations now not into the foot, tissues, or eyes causing calcification. The thyroid calls for magnesium. Hypothyroid troubles can be recommended at the identical time as a person would now not have enough magnesium. In order for the thyroid to function nicely the parathyroid, that is to your jaw line, have to uptake magnesium in order that weight loss plan C can be synthesized. The thyroid requires the calcium/magnesium ratio to be in right ratio and regularly this isn't always the case with critical calcium overload and not enough magnesium. Look at human beings as they age, do you spot human beings's bones turning into brittle or having a slump again? These are symptoms of calicfication collectively with bone spurs, arthritis, skin wrinkling, gout and the list goes on. Consider Trans-dermal Magnesium Oil Therapy, making use of it each day anywhere within the frame (except touchy regions) for six months to a three hundred and sixty five days. Reestablish the magnesium levels on your body with the shape of magnesium the body can understand and take in nicely. At first it will calm and detoxify your thyroid and frame. As time progresses, you may construct electricity, Jing, and stamina from the magnesium. In the start, use it at night time for restful sleep but as you assemble your lifestyles stress decrease lower back, comply with in advance within the day as you will check prolonged energy from it. This is an indicator you're returning notable magnesium tiers to your frame. If burning or stinging occurs, you need to dilute the magnesium oil with a 5:1 ratio (distilled water to magazine oil). Otherwise in that heavy attention, the body received't uptake it nicely. Or buy magnesium flakes and create your very own answer with distilled water. This will prevent cash. But honestly it ought to no longer sting your pores and pores and skin or cause infection, if it does there is probably fungus beneath the pores and pores and skin. Over time your pores and pores and skin will develop robust as you establish right magnesium/calcium ratios and exchange the intestine biome to ninety five% appropriate micro organism via probiotics and cultured food.

*Dr Group's Oxy Powder is Ozonated Magnesium so this is very useful for alkalinity throughout cleaning.

A look at about fats & weight loss:

For every greater pound of body weight there may be a diploma of infection in some unspecified time in the future of the device. This is because pollution are stored at some level in the body in fat, mainly heavy metals. This is one cause I significantly advocate going via the entire frame cleanse I shared with you, because of the reality as quick due to the fact the metals and the parasites the thyroid can feature to regulate your hormonal device and weight reduction begins offevolved to appear effortlessly. You start to appearance more more youthful and most significantly sense lively and enthusiastic about existence. The body isn't always afraid to permit bypass of the fat. The organs are unfold out and the pollutants can effectively go out . Your concept patterns now help your our our bodies healing and so it genuinely feels safe to permit pass of unneeded weight. The thyroid has been detoxed and reset, allowing it to feature with more electricity and vigor. Over time you need to look improvements as you improve your manner of lifestyles and live constant alongside side your cleaning physical sports.

In a Nutshell:

Your body has essential filters that require cleansing in order for the body's personal self-recovery mechanism to kick in.

Cleaning the precept filters out on a everyday basis will help each device artwork better, together with the thyroid, a part of the endocrine device.

We are hit with pollutants daily from air, food, water, and environment.

Start with the colon, then the liver/gallbladder, then the kidneys (when you have most important kidney troubles start with the kidneys first then do liver/gallbladder flush).

Once the precept channels are open once more, bear in mind a parasite and heavy metallic cleanse, this could in addition boost the burden off your thyroid and clean it out of particulates that have probable gotten lodged in it via poisonous compounds. It's rather advise to hold on to this step as parasites and heavy metals are in our environment, air, and water.

Magnesium is deficient in anyone and we must re-set up healthy degrees on the cellular level for proper thyroid feature and over all fitness/anti-growing old and immunity.

Weight loss is done resultseasily as a smooth, nourished frame comes forth and a upgraded manner of existence is followed.

Now that we have taken a have a take a look at the primary organ filters, we are able to circulate at once to the subsequent segment, mobile movement.

Try DIY methods. For Example:

Teeth Cleaning: A clean solution is Aluminum Free Baking Soda, Solar Dried Pink Salt, & plant primarily based MSM crystals. Mix collectively and store in a glass jar. Put a small quantity in your tooth brush and lightly polish your enamel. Add essential oils if you want for greater immunity.

To smooth the mouth and pull extra pollutants consider oil pulling with sesame or coconut oil. Add critical oils for extra anti-microbial energy. Take 2 Tbs of exceptional oil and graceful in mouth for up to twenty mins. This practice will lighten the load of pollution in the mouth assisting all talents of the body to artwork optimally. Treat your teeth like precious gems as they are connected to all components of your frame.

Shampoo: Experiment with apple cider vinegar, homemade shampoo or investigate agencies like Morrocco Method or Living Libations if you don't mind making an funding some cash in this place. For me, it's a pleasure to useful useful resource the ones agencies as they have got our excellent health in thoughts. As we consciously pick out those type of methods, our frame responds lower back with love and health. Setting a while aside to take a warm bathtub with vital oils and magnesium flakes facilitates calm the body and detoxify. Why no longer show your frame how a good deal you respect it? That appreciation will come again tenfold within the manner of extremely good health and a greater youthful glow.

Speaking of critical oils, the ones are plant capsules which may be here to help our our our bodies. When we get wild crafted crucial oils, we invoke the plant state's intelligence to assist in restoring our health. In this situation, the tremendous critical oil for restoring the thyroid is Green Myrtle. Green myrtle is an elixir of the gods. In Kurt Schnaubelt Ph.D's ebook, The Healing Intelligence of Essential Oils, he recommends this oil as a effective elixir for thyroid fitness. Rubbing this on the thyroid every day can create a wholesome immune reaction, because the plant's intelligence goes to paintings. I've placed no other important oils like that of Living Libations with regards to the purest high potency oils. Healing the body, I don't spare any charge on low amazing oils that are not of a immoderate fine. Consider this green myrtle and practice to a body pores and pores and pores and skin brush for lymphatic uptake. With the plant important oils, we supply the plant intelligence into our our bodies, reminding us of the oneness of lifestyles and the way all matters help us to heal. One of the outstanding topical meals for the thyroid and the remedy of a disease in the thyroid may be adaptogenic plant crucial oils. An adaptogen works like this: if some thing is out of stability, the intelligence of the herb or plant works its magic to heal and shield the goal organ/gland over time. For instance, if the thyroid is overactive it is going into calm it down and restore the gland. The following are my suggestions on the way to apply the myrtle oil.

First, make sure the deliver is ideal. It doesn't make an entire lot of revel in to collect a plant oil grown with pesticides, diluted or grown with out reverence. Remember, this is meals for the frame as well, it's without a doubt topical meals. So we can use a skin brush and upload a pair drops of the critical oil to our palm and brush the bristles of the pores and pores and skin brush over the oil. Next, begin at your ft and paintings the brush within the path of the coronary coronary heart all around the ground region of the body. When you get to the chest, neck, and face you could want to apply a face pores and skin brush and depart it without crucial oils. You also can take a drop of myrtle and positioned it at once at the thyroid and rub down the neck and throat vicinity. This is simply accurate to get things transferring and stimulate the lymph. Plants are a completely sensible species. They are proper here as our courses, treatment, and assistants in the aware journey. Spend time with them, experience their treatment, and get to realize them higher.

Medicinal Tea Brews for the Thyroid:

Ashwaganda - Adaptogen

Holy Basil - Adaptogen

Astragalus -Immunity Boost

Nettle - plenty of nourishing vitamins and iodine

Utilize a pleasant fat to strength the herbs into your gadget. Coconut oil is a tremendous preference right right here as it enables nourish the thyroid, or ghee, uncooked cultured pastured butter, or styrian gold pumpkin seed oil. If you don't digest fat nicely upload in a few sunflower lecithin powder to emulsify the fat or supplement with lipase enzymes to interrupt it down.

Other Nutritional Sources of Iodine:

Incorporate some one of a kind immoderate iodine plant meals. One of my all-time favorites are calendula plant life. You may additionally even wild harvest these yourself and they may be first rate for growing a medicinal tea. Remember we are what we devour, and wild plant life show off wild, natural beauty. Phi is embedded in all dwelling plant species. You can see the Fibonacci series in the ones flowers. This signature promotes lifestyles and the extra we consume topics in this healthy, lifestyles giving nation the extra we exude our true blue print. The word human translates to Light Eater (Hue - Light, Man - Eater).

Simply pass online and get a bulk of calendula flowers, as they'll be rich in iodine. Soak them in water within the sunlight hours for 7 hours and you've were given a nourishing solar tea. Try making a few warm temperature tea with them as properly. Nourish your light frame.

Another outstanding way to get your iodine via plant belongings are nettles. I get my sparkling nettles from a nearby forager. Add those to soups, smoothies, and other yummy recipes. They have an abundance of minerals too. When they may be no longer in season I often make nettle tea from the dry leaf which you can purchase online.

And, thru the way, some thing coconut you'll need to start loving if you don't already!

Coconut oil and coconut butter are marvel foods for the thyroid. It is a saturated fats and particularly strong, because of this that it gained't move rancid without issue, the liver does now not have oxidative pressure from this oil and the thyroid can use it fast which lets in sell a faster metabolism. Contrary to a few schools of concept, this form of fat is applied fast with the useful resource of the body for electricity and isn't always saved as extra fats.

Blood Sugar Levels moreover definitely impact the immune device and the fitness of your frame. Keeping blood glucose underneath eighty is a tremendous purpose. When those ranges rise to round 100 twenty, peripheral nerve damage begins to take location so stay with whole meals. There are devices you may buy to test blood glucose, however I experience that harming the body automatically thru pricking isn't smart interaction with our bio subject. If you put into impact the Body Ecology Principles and stay at the ketogenic (burning ketone's for electricity in place of glucose) component of things you may understand on the same time as you are in most desirable blood glucose variety by way of the usage of monitoring how you enjoy (elevated heart charge, jitters, mind fog might be symptoms of both improved blood sugar levels or mycotoxins from meals). Learn a way to gas your self with superior octane gasoline with the aid of manner of the use of ingesting meals that growth your life strain and immunity.

When the our bodies insulin is going up, the thyroid can reason an vehicle-immune response. Also, the hormones end up out of stability every time insulin receives too immoderate. It might not appear like an hassle however it absolutely changes the sport even as you maintain this in check with diet and way of existence picks. Keeping blood sugar levels in test is also a remarkable anti-growing vintage technique.

If you're overweight this might be going to do wonders for slimming you down. Grains, pasta, and all processed meals jack your stress hormones. Stick to a whole, non-processed ingredients diet plan approach.

Chapter 9: Good Thyroid Nutrition

You are what you devour—or in order that they are saying. That's why it's so vital to be aware of your diet, especially when you have a persistent state of affairs on the facet of thyroid sickness. The meals you pick out out will have a fantastic impact at the way you experience, in addition to how a whole lot weight you benefit (or lose). This financial smash gives some strategies for clever consuming when you have thyroid illness.

BASIC NUTRITION

Eating well is one of the cornerstones of tremendous fitness. But sadly, maximum American diets in recent times are a ways from maximum useful. They are weighted down with excessive-fats comfort food, extra sugar, and too many energy from huge quantities. To make subjects worse, mealtimes for lots human beings have end up erratic and uncommon, with too many food eaten on the run.

The truth is the food you select and the way you consume must make a large distinction on your fitness. On a every day foundation, they could have an effect on the manner you sense, how well you sleep, and the manner active you are. Over time, they will be capable of have an effect for your danger to grow to be overweight or obese and your vulnerability to intense diseases. To assist you are making smarter alternatives, it lets in to have a elegant understanding of primary vitamins.

Carbohydrates

Low carb. High carb. You pay attention hundreds about carbohydrates in recent times. Carbohydrates are your body's number one deliver of strength and are available two bureaucracy: clean and complicated. Simple carbs are the ones determined absolutely in fruits, greens, and milk, as well as meals that comprise touchy sugars, that have been processed to extract the natural sucrose discovered in vegetation for a sweeter flavor.

Simple carbs wreck down unexpectedly, supplying you with a quick burst of power. Healthy smooth carbs include end result, greens, and coffee-fats dairy products. Unhealthy smooth carbs encompass cakes, cookies, crackers, sugary cereals, and snack food. Rice, potatoes, and corn are also clean carbs that a few recommend retaining off.

Complex carbohydrates are considered the healthier carbs and are manufactured from starches and fiber determined sincerely in legumes, grains, and vegetables. Starch is located in the garage structures of flowers, collectively with wheat, oats, potatoes, beans, and lentils. In the frame, starches destroy down into smooth sugars but achieve this more slowly than the clean carbs do.

Fiber, however, can not be digested within the belly and transformed into smooth sugars. That's because of the reality people lack the enzyme required to interrupt it down. Instead of being taken up by means of your body for energy, fiber is excreted, a fact that has made it a powerhouse in treating and relieving digestive troubles. A extra extended speak on fiber seems later on this economic break.

To maximize your fitness, eat a mild amount of complex carbs, a good way to assist maintain levels of cholesterol down and decrease weight gain. Limit simple carbs to give up end result and vegetables, which supply different wholesome vitamins. Try to cut back on your consumption of carbs composed regularly of sensitive sugars. These consist of cakes, cookies, crackers, sweet, ice cream, potato chips, sweetened sugars and juices, and maximum snack food. Some humans, like Dr. Friedman, keep in mind in and practice a low-carbohydrate weight-reduction plan. Dr. Friedman tries to keep away from all risky smooth carbs and also minimizes complicated carbs. You need to talk for your medical doctor approximately the great meals for you.

Protein

Foods rich in protein supply the body with the amino acids had to bring together, repair, and maintain frame tissues. When your frame doesn't get sufficient carbohydrates or fat, it turns to protein for strength. Protein is found in meat, eggs, legumes, seeds, nuts, soybeans, and tofu. Getting enough protein, that is normally no longer a problem within the American diet, ensures healthy muscle and tissues.

Although protein has prolonged been related to constructing muscle, it absolutely doesn't assemble muscle power or duration with the aid of itself. Only through combining protein with strength schooling can there be any muscle building. But do not forget, any extra protein you consume is stored as fat and not burned as strength.

One of the great topics approximately protein is that it lets in you revel in whole so you are much less in all likelihood to overeat. In human beings with hypo- or hyperthyroidism who've an extended urge for food, protein can also help calm the urge to devour and decrease any excess weight gain.

Fats

Fats have been demonized for the usa of a's weight issues. But in truth, fats is an important nutrient, critical to the mind and worried gadget. It is also the substance that lends cheesecake its clean, creamy texture and makes macaroni and cheese so wealthy and appealing.

The trouble with fats is its high caloric density. Unlike carbohydrates and protein, which deliver 4 electricity regular with gram, fats gives a whopping nine electricity in step with gram, making it the maximum concentrated form of electricity. Fat is to be had in four essential paperwork:

Monounsaturated Fats

Monounsaturated fats that get up certainly in avocados and olive oil are the healthiest fats.

Unsaturated Fats

Polyunsaturated fats are drinks found in vegetable oils, inclusive of safflower, sunflower, and corn, and aren't as healthy as monounsaturated fat. However, omega-3 fatty acids, determined in fish, are a healthful form of polyunsaturated fats.

Saturated Fats

These are the harmful fat that clog arteries and raise the chance of coronary heart sickness. These are sturdy at room temperature and are to be had from meat, complete dairy food, butter, and palm and coconut oils.

Trans Fatty Acids

These fat aren't determined in nature but are produced whilst oils are hydrogenated to reason them to stable at room temperature. These are located in all processed components, together with breakfast cereals, frozen pancakes, potato chips, crackers, and cookies. They're additionally determined in margarine and shortening.

The hassle with fat takes place while you devour an excessive amount of of it. The dense strength make it a brief and surefire manner to advantage weight. And too much of the harmful forms of fat can cause fitness issues, inclusive of coronary heart infection, diabetes, and positive cancers.

VITAMINS AND MINERALS

Mother constantly stated to take your vitamins, and she became proper—

vitamins and minerals deliver the frame with critical substances that maximize our fitness and body competencies. While nutrients and minerals do not deliver the frame with power, they do assist facilitate reactions that produce energy from the components you eat.

The phrase nutrients is associated with precise fitness, but you could get too much of an great trouble. Certain vitamins in extra can purpose fitness issues. Too a exquisite deal nutrition A, for example, can reason complications, dry pores and pores and skin, joint ache, and liver harm. Excess niacin, a B food regimen, can purpose flushed pores and pores and skin, rashes, and liver harm. Too a exceptional deal nutrients E can sell bleeding.

Vitamin A, as an instance, guards in opposition to infections, even as weight-reduction plan D permits make more potent bones. And you apprehend that iodine, a mineral, is critical to the manufacturing of thyroid hormone.

When you've got thyroid disorder, positive minerals and elements play a larger characteristic in the way you feel and the way nicely your medicines artwork. The rest of this economic disaster zeroes in on particular dietary elements that could have an effect to your fitness and well-being.

Iodine

Iodine occurs evidently in seafood, seaweed, and kelp—mainly plant life and animals placed in saltwater. The mineral is likewise placed in milk, meat, spinach, and eggs. The bulk of it within the American diet, but, comes from iodized salt.

The encouraged each day dietary allowance of iodine for adults is a hundred fifty mcg. In pregnant women, the quantity goes up to 220 mcg. And in girls who're breast-feeding, it will increase to 290 mcg. But relaxation assured. Getting those quantities is notably clean. All it takes to attain the RDA for adults is half a teaspoon of iodized salt.

Too Much Iodine

People who have wholesome thyroids can devour as lots as ten times extra iodine than what's advocated and nonetheless be exquisite. But in people who have a thyroid problem, an excessive amount of iodine is dangerous. Excess iodine can honestly inhibit the manufacturing of thyroid hormone, causing goiter and hypothyroidism. And when you have already had been given hyperthyroidism, extra iodine ought to make your signs and signs and symptoms and signs worse.

Too Little Iodine

The traditional U.S. Eating habitual these days is wealthy in iodine. In fact, it's more apt to have an excessive amount of iodine than it's far to be in quick supply. Since the Twenties, america of the united states has cherished a plentiful supply of iodized salt.

Worldwide, however, the shortage of iodine is a common hassle, and it remains a massive public fitness trouble on a global scale.

But if you're on a low-sodium weight-reduction plan, you will be at chance for no longer getting sufficient iodine. This might be more likely if you live inland and do now not eat seafood. Without enough iodine, your frame can not produce the thyroid hormone it wishes, and you will be at risk for hypothyroidism and goiter. Most multivitamins comprise enough iodine, so in case you are concerned about iodine deficiency, you can take a multivitamin. And don't forget, thyroid medicinal capsules, consisting of levothyroxine and Cytomel, include a massive quantity of iodine, so if you are on thyroid hormone alternative, you do not need to worry approximately your iodine consumption.

Soy

Asian cultures have stated approximately soy for years, but it's a pretty new meals to the American weight loss plan. In present day years, soy has emerged as a nutritional powerhouse, manner to analyze that have associated it to fighting contamination. Isoflavones, substances discovered in soy, are stated to assist fight breast most cancers, tame the new flashes of menopause, restrict the bone loss that takes place in postmenopausal girls, and decrease your threat of coronary heart disease by using the usage of lowering cholesterol. In essence, soy acts as a phytoestrogen, or plant estrogen.

But a have a look at in early 2006, in the mag Circulation, furnished a greater humble view of this wonder bean. The take a look at located that isoflavones had only a moderate impact on lowering LDL, the horrible ldl cholesterol. The researchers additionally decided no massive consequences on HDL, the exceptional ldl cholesterol; triglycerides; and blood stress.

In addition, soy had little effect on warm flashes and bone loss in postmenopausal women. They moreover located no evidence that soy can also need to treat or prevent positive cancers, which embody breast most cancers. But the researchers did no longer reduce price the benefits of excessive excellent soy merchandise, which might be excessive in protein, fiber, vitamins, and minerals.

Where Is Soy?

Soy is a bean found in meals as severa as tofu; tempeh; soymilk; soy sauce; and miso, a soybean paste. The pleasure over soy has unleashed a tidal wave of new soy merchandise, which includes soy burgers, soy shakes, and soy cereals. People also use tofu to make chili, lasagna, and cakes.

Troubles with Soy

In people who have hypothyroidism, too much soy can irritate a thyroid hassle. The isoflavones observed in soy can increase TSH tiers, causing an increase in hormone requirements and the capacity for goiter. In ladies, greater soy can cause menstrual irregularities that can cause infertility.

I pay attention some factor amazing about soy every day. What am I purported to believe?

Nutrition news appears to be all the time evolving, and simplest nice truths have emerged approximately pick factors, for example, saturated fats are terrible. Take any breaking facts with a grain of salt and a healthful dose of skepticism. And inside the meantime, stick with the old adage: Everything cautiously.

Soy can also inhibit absorption of thyroid medicines. So if you want to devour soy, ensure you don't eat it across the equal time you take your thyroid remedy. Instead, you want to wait at the least four hours after taking your thyroid medicinal drug before ingesting some detail that includes soy.

Caffeine

Every morning, you awaken feeling tired and slow till you get that morning cup of joe. If you're like many humans, you want a jolt of caffeine to get you moving, be it a cup of coffee or tea. According to a test in 2004, 87 percentage of adults and 76 percent of youngsters have caffeine of their each day diets, this is higher than the eighty percent and forty three percent, respectively, determined in 1977.

The reality is, caffeine is a drug, a prison stimulant placed in numerous food and medications that may have profound consequences at the applicable concerned device. Over the years, caffeine has been accused of contributing to a number of illnesses and conditions, however no hyperlink has ever been confirmed.

What is plain is that caffeine stimulates your frame's production of adrenaline, one of the combat-or-flight hormones. Although the initial surge of adrenaline offers you an power enhance, its next decline motives a crash that can reason carb cravings and overeating. Caffeine moreover reasons a transient rise in blood stress and further commonplace urination, which could growth your excretion of calcium. In more, caffeine can motive insomnia, tension, and coronary coronary heart palpitations.

Where's the Buzz?

Caffeine is located in some of elements, along facet coffee, tea, mild beverages, and chocolate. It is likewise placed in electricity liquids, caffeinated water, weight loss program aids, bloodless treatments, migraine medicinal capsules, and sure menstrual pain relievers.

Restrict Caffeine

People who've thyroid sickness need to be cautious about consuming too much caffeine. In humans who've hyperthyroidism, too much caffeine can exacerbate your signs and make you experience even greater nervous, aggravating, and jittery. It also can worsen any coronary heart irregularities.

If you've got weight issues associated with hypothyroidism, you'll be tempted to attempt diet plan aids that include caffeine. Caffeine's stimulant effects do appear to in short beautify weight loss. But the outcomes on weight consist of a charge, specifically tension, tension, and sleep troubles. In turn, the lack of splendid sleep can stimulate your urge for food, that would sabotage any weight reduction efforts. The backside line is that this: Try to devour as little caffeine as possible.

Goitrogens

In healthful human beings, ingesting an abundance of quit quit end result and veggies has been touted as a key way to keep illnesses like coronary coronary coronary heart sickness, most cancers, and diabetes at bay. Fruits and veggies also are celebrated as key additives for wholesome weight reduction and manipulate. But in people who have thyroid disorder, too pretty a few high quality stop give up end result and vegetables may additionally moreover furthermore have a negative impact.

These food are known as goitrogens, a word derived from the time period goiter. Goitrogens stimulate the formation of goiters. These food block the effects of an enzyme referred to as thyroid peroxidase, which is needed for the manufacturing of thyroid hormone.

Types of Goitrogens

Many cruciferous greens are goitrogens. These encompass broccoli, cauliflower, Brussel sprouts, cabbage, turnips, and rutabagas. But special food which incorporates spinach, strawberries, radishes, peaches, millet, soy merchandise, corn, candy potatoes, carrots, peanuts, and walnuts also are taken into consideration goitrogens.

Limit Goitrogens

People who don't have thyroid sickness can enjoy the ones food with out a high-quality deal hassle, however in people with thyroid troubles, the ones goitrogens are probable complex, particularly if eaten in extra. To advise which you surrender those healthful meals, but, seems counterintuitive to suitable fitness, thinking about all the nutrients that the ones meals encompass. A better opportunity is to eat those meals carefully and at a substantially steady quantity from sooner or later to the subsequent. You need to moreover make certain to get your TSH examined frequently. Also, these meals are plenty much less volatile to people who have ok iodine intake, making them an entire lot much less damaging to people living within the United States.

Calcium

Unfortunately, most girls nowadays do not get sufficient calcium in their diets. They drink soda as opposed to milk, refuse to eat leafy green veggies, and don't hassle with a supplement. In truth, the not unusual American weight-reduction plan includes awesome about 500 to 750 mg of calcium.

Although most of the calcium in your frame is for your bones, the mineral moreover lets in muscle tissue to agreement, blood to clot, and your coronary heart to overcome. If you don't get sufficient on your weight loss plan, your body will take what it needs out of your bones, which will purpose your bones to become thin. That's why true sufficient calcium consumption is so vital.

If you're involved approximately bone fitness, lessen lower again on alcohol.

Consuming extra than seven oz.Of alcohol per week—the identical of 1 drink consistent with day—reduces bone density. Because alcohol affects your balance and coordination, it'll increase the chance of falls and hip fractures. Alcohol is likewise excessive in empty electricity—seven energy everyday with gram.

This thinning of bone is exacerbated in ladies with hyperthyroidism because of the stimulation of osteoclasts through the usage of the extra thyroid hormone.

Where's the Calcium?

Most of the calcium you get comes from your food regimen. Good belongings of dietary calcium encompass low-fat milk, yogurt, and cheese. An eight-ounce glass of skim milk, for example, gives 298 mg of calcium, on the same time as an 8-ounce serving of yogurt gives you 415 mg. An ounce of Swiss cheese affords 219 mg. You can also discover calcium in fortified orange juice, canned fish with in shape for human intake bones, leafy inexperienced veggies, and tofu.

In addition, calcium is determined in dietary dietary supplements and multivitamins. But maximum multivitamins do no longer have enough calcium to meet your each day desires.

Get Your Calcium

Women with thyroid illness want to pay precise hobby to their calcium intake, specifically within the occasion that they've hyperthyroidism. According to the National Institutes of Health, in case you're over age fifty and taking estrogen, you want 1,000 mg of calcium constant with day. If you're over fifty and not taking estrogen, you need 1,500 mg an afternoon. Women between the a while of twenty-five and fifty need to get 1,000 mg an afternoon.

Although it's better to get your calcium from food property, opportunities are you received't fulfill your necessities, so most ladies want to take a supplement, too. When selecting a complement, make sure to check the label for the quantity of elemental calcium in it. To maximize absorption, take dietary nutritional supplements with meals or orange juice. If you take more than 750 mg of calcium supplements in step with day, take one dose in the morning and each other in advance than bedtime when you do not forget that your body can soak up only so much calcium at a time.